Are You Healthy Enough For Sex?

Sex May Not Be For Everyone

Guide to Knowing the Risks and Benefits of Sex.

"A true warrior only fights the
battle he can win."
(Sun Tze, The Art of War)

" Know one's enemy well and in a
100 battles you will merge
victoriously."
(Sun Tze, The Art of War)

Are You Healthy Enough for Sex?

Copyright © 2015 by Dr. Angelo Isom, ND, CHS, MQT

Visit my website for future updates, products and services. Phone consults are available via appointments as well.

www.lifeishealing.com

www.harmonizingfist.com

ISBN-13: 978-1511817097
ISBN-10: 1511817097

Medical Disclaimer

The information provided in this book is designed to provide helpful information on the subjects discussed. This book is not meant to be used, nor should it be used, to diagnose or treat any medical condition. For diagnosis or treatment of any medical problem, consult your own physician. The publisher and author are not responsible for any specific health or allergy needs that may require medical supervision and are not liable for any damages or negative consequences from any treatment, action, application or preparation, to any person reading or following the information in this book. References are provided for informational purposes only.

Brief Biography of Dr. Angelo Isom, ND, CHS, MQT

Dr. Angelo Isom is a graduate of New York University, Columbia University, Georgia State University and Clayton College of Natural Healing. He holds several degrees in various fields including psychology, philosophy, teaching methods, education and naturopathy and numerous other certifications. Dr. Isom has written and published his first book on male sexual health and well being entitled, "The Sexual Warrior Within,". Apart from writing, he is also a male health advisor, martial arts lineage holder and avid researcher.

Dr. Isom's experiences in healing encompass multiple areas of research and study. Some of these areas include acupuncture, yoga, internal martial arts, qi gong, energy healing, human sexuality, western and eastern herbs, diet and nutrition.

Dr. Isom has been fortunate to study cultural healing methods and herbs while visiting such countries as Brazil, Mexico's Yucatan Peninsula, Haiti, Jamaica and Puerto Rico. Dr. Isom is CEO and director of Life is Healing, a holistic wellness ministry. Over the years, he has counseled many clients seeking to achieve optimal fitness and health.
Dr. Isom's approach to healing and rejuvenation focuses upon the cultivation of vital energy of qi, grounding, internal cleansing, eating according to the seasons, mind/body balance, and lifestyle.

Reviews

"Dr. Isom has done an excellent job in showcasing sexual issues that plague men of all ages today. Men can now feel optimistic in choosing a solution that is right for them. I highly recommend that every man young and old read the Sexual Warrior Within. Women should definitely buy this book for their lover or husband"
---- C. Blackburn, Health and Wellness Coach

"Finally, man's modern day natural guide for Herbal Viagra without the side effects. Read and study this book and you will be on the right track."
---- C. Parks, Nurse LPN and Holistic Healing Counselor and Advocate.

"After following Dr. Isom's teachings on qi gong and taking natural herbs I have experienced more skeletal flexibility and internal organ strength. The information in the Sexual Warrior Within has improved my health, sex life, and mental attitude."
David T. --- retired railroad worker and robust 65 year young.

"Being a media professional is demanding both physically and mentally. I began a health regimen of internal martial arts, qigong, and herbal supplement's under Dr. Isom. My health has improved since I began, I am better able to focus and work at my best level."
- --Tau Justice, Southside Media, LLC.

" It is easy to tell that Dr. Isom is very passionate about this subject. He has dedicated a great deal of his life to help men regain their confidence and sense of manhood. With this book, men will not only have the knowledge of what to do if they are having various male issues, but they will also have the power to prevent these issues in the first place. I am very excited about the knowledge that Dr. Isom has brought forth. This book is really a game changer." **--- Crystal Lawrence, MBA**

"This book is a must read for both men and women. For men, it is a handbook for healthy living and sexual vitality. With this tool, men will no longer be dependent upon sexual wellness or stamina drugs. Dr. Isom's book provides freedom of choice. Stamina and endurance can be achieved naturally free of drugs without damaging side effects. Every woman that has a man in her life should also be knowledgeable about the options presented to men through this book. Women are key motivators to their mates; and in return, can encourage their partners to follow the lifestyle changes that are presented. In summary, this is everyone's book." **ChieStine Lawrence, Computer Technology Engineer and IT Consultant.**

Preface

This book was developed out of the need to consolidate my personal research and insightful discoveries about human sexuality and performance issues often encountered by men. Many of my notes were often scattered across my work desk either buried in old folders, internet files or simply lost due to my failure to document properly. One day, I thought wouldn't it be great if most of my research could be consolidated in one reliable sustainable place. It was then that I decided on placing them into a book format for retrieval. Getting started and organizing information seemed to be quite intimidating for someone like me that usually post information anywhere for convenience. After hours, days and weeks of cleaning up, evaluating and reorganizing mounds of information and data, I reconstructed my archive. The next big step was outlining and updating my research with current research.

Gradually everything became clear and I began to process my notes in a systematic concise way. Imposing discipline upon myself to write daily turned out to be one of several the key factors for my success. After 6 months of continuous writing I still had to overcome numerous problems with editing, copywriting, ISBN and marketing. In the end the final path was made clear and worth the journey.

Dedication

This book is dedicated to all the members of my immediate and extended family for their kindness, inspiration and devotion. I would like to extend special thanks to all of my martial arts students, family and friends, especially Eric Graham, Tau Justice for there support in convincing me that I should write this book and have it published. Special thanks to Crystal and ChieStine Lawrence for assisting me in the promotion of my book by creating the lifeishealing.com website and for their dedication and support of my business endeavors.

 Last but not least, an enduring thanks to Cathy Blackburn for her support on the design of the book cover and encouragement. This book is also dedicated to all men who struggle day to day to be the man that they were meant to be. All men who want to preserve their health and maintain healthy testosterone levels should read and study this book. A healthy sex life is well worth pursuing. Many men struggle quietly every day to be healthy, loving, romantic and sexy but often encounter many obstacles. Settling for impotency or being celibate is not an option or forced choice.

The sexual warrior within each man does not want to lay down arms and surrender to the emasculating process of modern living. Some men simply accepted defeat or allowed themselves to become easily disillusioned.

 It is my goal to recruit them once again and harness the sexual warrior within. It is my goal that the reader will greatly benefit from the knowledge and practical strategies given in this book to preserve and recover their sexual lifestyle.

Table of Content

The Mind / Body Connection/Affirmations

Many men tend to overlook the importance of the mind body connection when it comes to sex. Sex is not all physical in nature. This connection can have profound influence on a man's health, vitality and erectile power. Using positive affirmation daily can rewire your mental habits and subconscious beliefs to actually influence the biological processes of the entire body.

By regularly conditioning your mind with these affirmations you will encourage your body to send blood flow to your penis, strengthen the tissue and muscle in the pelvis, and naturally increase your sex drive. Thoughts are everything. The way we think empowers our daily actions and health. Thoughts definitely affect hormonal balance shifting us into high or low gear. When the word is spoken it is materialize as intent leading us to a specific course of action and outcome.

I encourage you not to underestimate the power of affirmations. When saying affirmations one must match the proper emotional element with it. Emotional content combine with a directive affirmation leads to personal manifested power.

Affirmations without an emotional root are impotent. Review the following affirmations and decide which of them is applicable. Choose well.

" Change your thoughts and you change the world"
                                    - Norman Vincent Peale

AFFIRMATIONS FOR SEXUAL POWER

Present Tense Affirmations
I am sexually confident
I am a great lover
I am a powerful sexual being
I am in touch with my deepest sexual nature and desire
I always please my partner
I am open to new sexual experiences
I am secure in my body and celebrate its sexuality
I express my deepest sexual needs
I am a sexually confident man
My penis is strong and hard
My body directs blood flow to my penis
My penis has excellent circulation
My erections are long lasting
My partner is turned on by my hardness
I am free from worry and stress
I am revitalizing my penile tissue with the power of my mind
I always achieve erection
My penis is healthy

Future Tense Affirmations
I will unleash my sexual confidence
I will express my sexual nature
I am developing magnetic sexual power
I am becoming sexually confident
My sexual confidence is growing
I am overcoming my sexual insecurities
I am starting to explore my wildest fantasies
I will provide immense sexual pleasure to my partner
I am becoming a highly skilled lover
I am noticing my partner is turned on by my sexual confidence

My Personal Quotes and Thoughts

Sex is only good as it is leveraged

All men have the right to life, liberty and the pursuit of sex.

Men must say no to celibacy and yes to orgasm.

Next to life itself sex is the one of the greatest gifts in the world.

Men are at risk today and tomorrow when it comes to a healthy a sex life. Sex can not be taken for granted.

The notion of manhood is constantly being redefined.

The world is becoming more feminine everyday.

Having a normal healthy testosterone levels is considered an endangered event.

Your life is your sex and sex is your life.

Without dopamine there is no lust. Without lust there is no sex.

Men with low testosterone levels are easy to control and manipulate.

"Live Your Life by Design and Not Fate"

You only miss 100% of the women you don't pursue and the conquest you leave to fate.

Every man is a sexual warrior.

Being sexually active is a good index of health

Without strong male sexual energy a nation cannot secure its future and survive upheavals.

The right of passage to manhood has been deleted from our culture and is no longer treated as a right.

I am the lord and master of my bedroom.

Keep sex alive!

Homo-sapien equals Homo-erectus from a sexual point of view.

Instead of focusing on the woman you want try focusing your time and energy on the woman that wants you.

Don't be a man that needs a woman but rather the man that a woman needs.
Without life there is no sex.
Without sex there is no life.

All Men Should Strive to Become an Alpha Male = I (AM)

Being an alpha male, (AM) has more to do with attitude than altitude or size. Simply put it's all about empowerment. An AM leads, direct, controls while achieving dominance over his dominion and sexual lifestyle. He utilizes all of his resources and dedicates himself to being 100% of the man he can be. The AM sets the standard for his right to passage into manhood. Most women are conditioned to desire, respect and fantasize about being ravished by a gentle AM. He literally tends to dominate the bedroom. Many women are taught to settle for an omega male, (OM) out of need or in exchange for modern day financial security. The OM is conditioned to lose, settle and be easily dominated by both men and other women. Men that are controlled by their wives are omega males.

Women in general are usually empathetic and tolerant of a man's shortcomings. Because of their enormous capacity for compassion and love, women tolerate an OM if he makes a commitment to care for her, raise and protect the family. Given this scenario and the pressures of social obligations, the notion of prioritizing a healthy sex life is usually reduced to the status of a secondary fantasy.

An alpha male can be defined as a winner who takes what he wants, maintains his conquest while being willing to pay the price to do so. Many of the world's formidable Alpha Males were also bold daring men of small physical stature. Some examples of these men, to name a few, could include Napoleon, Bruce Lee, and Geronimo.

Introduction

This book was written as a non technical guide with detailed explanation to help the reader better understand why and how the male sexual energy system works. Once understood, the reader will be better able to apply more appropriate strategies and interventions to help restore sexual vitality. Sexual energy manifests itself in more ways than just the all too familiar romantic interplay between man and woman or lust. It is by nature the creative potential energy that drives the artist, boxer or entrepreneur.

Sexual energy can manifest itself as the source of courage and commitment needed to start a new business or investment in a risky but profitable business venture. Simply put, it is the motivation and raw desire to succeed at a given task or goal leading to a more pleasurable outcome. All great men and leaders throughout history shared a common thread of heighten primal sexual energy transformed or transmuted into a specific goal.

This is why it is vital for all people to cultivate, preserve and protect their sexual energy. Our sexual energy can also have a profound impact on our daily health. Many studies have shown that sexual energy and health are often correlated. The key ingredients are often indicative of a good heart and robust circulation of blood and hormones.

Without health there is no sex. Without sex health does not thrive. Good sexual energy can save marriages, boost our immune system, improve prostate health, regulating a woman's menstrual cycle and sometimes even prevent wars.

It is my quest to sexually empower the average male by increasing awareness to multicultural and global alternatives integrated with modern wisdom. I commend those men who still want to engage in vigorous sexual activity but feel compromised by lack of health and poor lifestyle choices.

If you want to get your body and your sex life back on track, you'll find the tools and strategies you need to make it happen right here.

Many men fail to understand that there are indeed a plethora of solutions that are natural and noninvasive waiting to be discovered. Viagra free erections are still a reality worth pursing. The average male no longer needs to rely exclusively upon drugs such as Viagra and synthetic low testosterone gels highly publicized on TV commercials, radio and magazines. During ancient times if a warrior dropped his sword he could easily lose his life. The sword symbolized the warrior's manhood, ability to fight and preserve his freedom and sexual potency. Today the stakes are quite similar for modern man. The sword is now symbolic modern man's his genital and sexual potency.

Be aware that there are always constant threats looming in the background that can threaten one's manhood. If the sexual warrior drops his testosterone level and libido too low then he too could lose his sex life. All warriors should have an attitude of readiness and resolve to win and or survive any confrontation. A healthy sex life is worth fighting for. The sexual warrior should be dedicated to maintaining a healthy readiness status to engage in the art of lovemaking when ever confronted by a beautiful consensual woman.

It is nature and inner nature that will guide each man down the right path without risks of dangerous side effects and dependency upon synthetic aphrodisiacs. Many men simply do not realize that there is a daily ongoing battle raging within themselves trying to find that delicate balance of hormones, libido and erection power. Proper peripheral blood flow and testosterone levels can fluctuate from moment to moment and day-to-day.

Every metabolic process in the body must be timed correctly. The hormonal or endocrine system of the body can be compared to a car.

If the engine of a car is not tuned or timed properly, it will fail to crank or maintain combustion. Quite similar to the human body many of these internal processes are time sensitive. A more detailed explanation of these biochemical processes will be discussed later in the chapter on the Biology of Libido.

After much research on sexual energy, personal exploration and surveying of numerous personal testimonies, I became compelled to write this book. The gradual decline of both libido and sexual vigor should not be understood as a natural process of aging. This belief model is far from the truth especially when we compare modern man to the indigenous tribal communities of Latin America, Africa and Native Americans. These people are far healthier and robust in terms of fertility, libido and sexual energy. What are their secrets? How are these people able to remain in hormonal paradise? Many of these people live in close alliance with nature and continue to maintain sexual vigor well into their 90s.

Many ancient healing and sexual enhancement practices are often misunderstood or tabooed. The dawning of a new sexual revolution and renaissance that fosters enhancement, performance and true intimacy awaits the reader of this book. The science of present day knowledge and its modus operandi for improving male sexual potency is also analyzed in detail with regards to pros and cons. Men everywhere should no longer have to resort to sacrificing long term health for short term gains using conventional means. What we need today is a paradigm shift of thinking. This new model of thinking states that one can be physically fit at any age and be sexually active as well. Issues relating to sexual problems must be attacked from many angles using a variety of approaches such as testosterone supplements, ejaculation control, chemical avoidance, and estrogen reduction etc.

Chapter 1

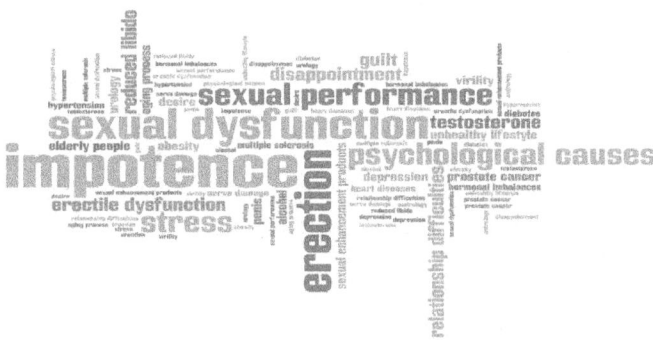

Age Related Sexual Decline in Male Sexual Performance

Sexual performance is probably the most common concern of both young and aging men as it relates to their health and relationships. The average man's sexual peak usually occurs around the age of 18. Due to poor diet and the stresses of modern living and unhealthy lifestyles significant declines in sexual performances can occur as early as 26 years of age. Most men began to notice a longer time needed to be aroused and to achieve a full erection. These problems can range from a less than firm erection, lower libido, decrease in sexual stamina and lower volume of ejaculation during orgasm.

As men age there is usually a drop in the production of hormones such as DHEA, testosterone and other related androgens or sex hormones. When men reach the age of 40 their testosterone level can decrease by 1% for each following year. Research clearly shows that about 20% of men in their 60s and 50% of men in their 80's have significantly reduced testosterone levels.

Testosterone is a key hormone in men's sexual function, aging-related decline in testosterone levels can have a negative impact on self-esteem and sexual performance. As sexual performance is closely related to men's overall health, factors that affect general health, such as anxiety, stress, and psychological factors, can also affect sexual performance. Fortunately, any decline associated with these factors can usually be reversed once the underlying causes are resolved.

There is a light at the end of this tunnel. Many of these symptoms of decline that are age-related can actually be reversed. What is most important and part of the solution is having a stress-free and active healthy lifestyle. Many men notice a distinct improvement in sexual performance and overall health when smoking, alcohol and recreational drug use are eliminated or kept to a minimum.

Low testosterone level can be medically treated by testosterone replacement therapy. The ultimate goal of this therapy is to increase serum levels of testosterone by means of injection, oral dosage and trans-dermal delivery of testosterone.

Testosterone replacement therapy can also be risky if one chooses this approach. Close monitoring of serum androgen levels should be done periodically by a qualified physician. The use of herbal extracts and formulations have clinically been shown to offer a more promising solution in reversing age-related decline in men.

Protodiocin is one of the active compounds found an herbal plant commonly known as tribulus terrestris. Tribulus clinically has been shown the ability to increase both the level of DHEA and testosterone in men. One clinical study on 15 men with decreased sexual performance indicated that nearly 90% of them treated with tribulus at 500 mg 3X daily for 60 days experience a significantly improved libido, ejaculation, and orgasm as compared to before the treatment. Protodioscin treatment resulted in significantly increased sex drive 33% of men after 30 days and in 80% of men after 60 days. Similarly, arousal improved in 53% of men after 30 days and 87% of men after 60 days. Orgasm sensation and ejaculate quality also improved significantly in 40% and 87% of men after 30 and 60 days.

In another clinical study, 60 non-diabetic men with and without erectile dysfunctions and 15 diabetic men with sexual performance problems were given protodioscin) at 3 x 250 mg per day for 3 weeks. The study found that in addition to increased DHEA levels in the treated group, the frequency of successful intercourse increased by 60%. In addition, an improved sense of well-being, improved sensation, erection, ejaculation, and orgasm were also reported by the treated men. In these and other clinical studies on tribulus protodioscin, there were no unwanted side effects or contraindications.

Tribulus Terrestris is slowly becoming a very popular herb. Unfortunately, not all commercially available tribulus contain the active ingredient protodioscin at the standardized level or dosage to produce results. A saponin level of 45% or higher is needed by most men to duplicate the same level of success as seen in the research studies.

References:

1. Morley, JE. Testosterone replacement in older men and women. J Gend Specif Med. 2001; 4:49-53

2. Viktorov I, Bozadjieva E, Protich M, et al. Pharmacological, pharmacokinetic, toxicological and clinical studies on protodioscin. 1994, IIMS Therapeutic Focus

3. Arsyad KM. Effect of protodioscin on the quantity and quality of sperms from males with moderate idiopathic oligozoospermia. Medika 22 (8): 614-618 (1996)

4. Adimoelja A and Ganeshan Adaikan P. Protodioscin from herbal plant Tribulus terrestris L improves the male sexual functions, probably via DHEA. Int. J. Impotence Research. 1997:9; Supp. 1

Chapter 2

Are You Healthy Enough to Have Sex?

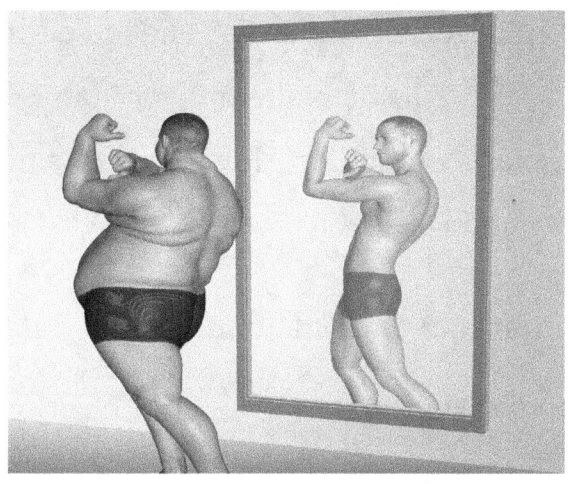

In India, Nepal, Tibet, China, and Japan, sexuality has long been regarded as both an art and a science worthy of detailed study and practice. Indeed, the Eastern view is that no learning is complete without a thorough knowledge of the sexual principles underlying all existence. Eastern metaphysical traditions make use of the mystery of sexuality as a means to the transcendental experience of Unity.

How healthy and physically fit are you? One should strive to be physically fit at any age. Many men tend to ignore the fact that having sex can be a very physically demanding act. During a typical erotic encounter there are dramatic physical changes that occurs n the body and brain. Both respiration and heart rate are normally elevated in anticipation along with increase in blood pressure. These bodily reactions are quite similar to what an athlete experiences just prior to competition or warm-ups. Other common reactions can also include muscle tension, perspiration, release of pheromones, nervousness, elevated stress hormones like cortisol, an increase of adrenaline and of course the release of testosterone.

Some of these physical changes are conducive for good sex and some of them can get in the way. Most athletes are very familiar with performance anxiety which can impair their ability. How much of a physical feat is having passionate intercourse?

Listed below areas that may indicate issues of sexual health:

1. Lack of self-confidence
2. Poor endurance
3. Lower back pain
4. Selfishness
5. Not interested in Sex
6. Depression
7. Unable to relax
8. Erectile dysfunction
9. No Energy
10. Weakness in knees
11. Easily angered

My new paradigm shift of thinking advocates that men should train for sex. Most people clearly recognize that in order to be good at sports you must train or workout on a regular basis. The physical training must fit the specific physical requirement of the sport. Why not do the same for sex? The term often used by coaches is called " Specificity of Training". One could almost easily equate having sex to trying out for high school sports. The requirements would be a full physical including heart monitoring and a permission slip from the doctor. For most men sex can easily represent the pinnacle of their manhood. Relax casual sex is by no means a strenuous physical endeavor

Studies have been conducted since 1984 that involved 10 married couples who were willing participants in a monitored lab setting. The key body markers were blood pressure, pulse and rate of oxygen consumption. The study revealed that normal causal sex poses little risk for both men and women. Most men today prefer to engage in all out intense passionate sex with women. When expectations for intense sex are high the physical demand also can increase. In previous experiment physical exertion during sex were measured in terms of metabolic equivalents or MET. One MET is also defined as 18.4 $Btu/h \cdot ft^2$, which is equal to the rate of heat energy produced per unit surface area of an average person seated at rest.

Based upon this system 1 met is equivalent to the amount of energy expended while sitting quietly. During the phase of casual relax sex when the man is on top having intercourse he spent on average 3.3 METS.

On the other hand, the study also showed that when the women were on top men expended on the average only 2.5 METS. A range of 1.1-2.9 is considered light intensity as compared to a range of 3.0 to 5.9 METS, the moderate intensity level. Another reference for MET values of activities can range from 0.9 (sleeping) to 23 (running at 22.5 km/h or a 4:17 mile pace).

It is quite evident that sex is different for everybody both physically and emotionally.

You may be surprised to learn what the simple definition of physical fitness. Physical Fitness is a measure of the body's ability to function efficiently and effectively in work and leisure activities, resist hypo-kinetic diseases (diseases from sedentary lifestyles), and to meet emergency situations. This definition was derived from decades of research by exercise physiologists and cardiologists.

The top 10 facets of physical fitness are adapted from sources that include the President Council on Fitness, Sports & Nutrition, Cross Fit, and the National Strength & Conditioning Association.

Physical Fitness # 1 <u>Body Composition</u>

Definition: The relative amount of fat, muscle, bone, and other vital parts of the body.

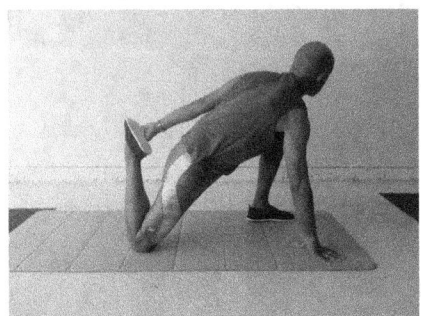

Copyright/ Dr. Isom

Measurement: Skin fold calipers, BIA, DEXA (see ways to measure body fat percentage)

Body Composition is always important. It is possible for an individual to have a high degree of fitness and still have excess body fat. Losing body fat while retaining lean muscle mass will improve all other physical attributes. Strength/power to weight ratio will also be improved along with other general health markers.

Physical Fitness # 2- <u>Strength</u>

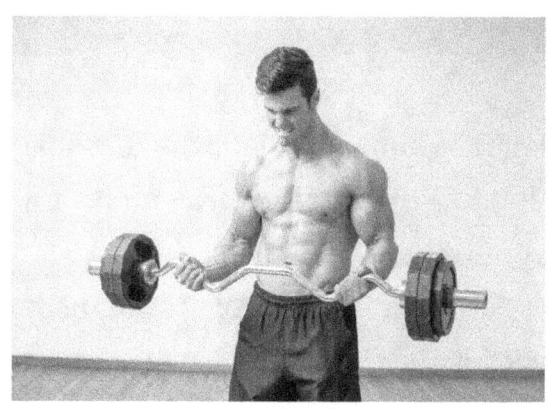

Strength is required to perform basic functional movements in our life like squatting, lunging, pushing, pulling, and bending are important in our everyday life. In addition, as we age muscle size and strength tend to decrease along with bone mass, which can be reversed with strength training. Measurement: Multiple tests must be completed to test more than one muscle group. Examples include max effort on exercises like the squat, bench press, or dead lift from 1-6 repetitions.

Physical Fitness #3 | <u>Cardiovascular Fitness</u>
Definition: Ability of the circulatory systems and respiratory systems to supply oxygen during sustained physical activity.
Measurement: VO2 Max Test, sub-maximal YMCA

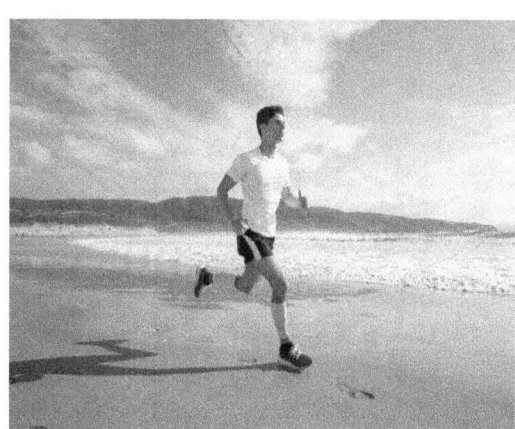

Significance: Cardiovascular exercises increase lung capacity so the heart does not have to work as hard to pump blood to the muscles. Respiration is important for overall heart health and prevention of lifestyle diseases.

Definition: Ability of the circulatory systems and respiratory systems to supply oxygen during sustained physical activity.

Measurement: VO2 Max Test, sub-maximal YMCA Step Test

Significance: An improved cardiovascular system increases lung capacity so the heart does not have to work as hard.

Physical Fitness #4 | <u>Flexibility</u>

Definition: The range of motion at a joint

Measurement: There is no specific test because there are many joints in the human body, but a range of stretches can identify flexibility like the sit and reach test, shoulder reach etc. Significance: The optimal range of motion about various joints has a direct effect on almost all other facets of physical fitness. For example, if one's hip flexors are tight, that can affect the ability to reach maximum speed, or perform agility drills at a high level.

For some flexibility is innate while others have to work hard to acquire it. Flexibility has to be approached gradually without strain and pain. A realistic expectation

of improving one's range of motion should be based upon correct stretching method, consistent routines and warm-ups.

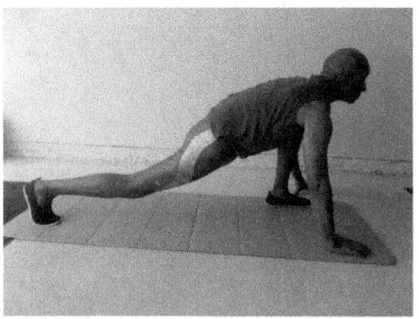

Physical Fitness #5 | <u>Muscular Endurance</u>

Definition: The ability of muscles to continue to perform repeated contractions.

Measurement: Given there is more than one major muscle group, testing muscular endurance requires testing each individual muscle, or group. Examples include maximum number of push-ups, sit-ups, pull-ups, and dips.

Significance: Performing repetitious physical activity such as gardening, raking leaves and washing your car are common activities that can improve endurance.

Health, Nutrition, and Wellness – Mental fitness, nutrition and wellness are also integral parts of optimal fitness. In fact, optimal fitness could never be achieved without adequate mental fitness and proper nutrition.

One should clearly understand why physical fitness is so important when it comes to being able to have good sex. Top priority should be given to fitness before considering the use of Viagra/Cialis or Low T topical gels to boost overall wellness and libido.

Again I pose the question, how much of a physical feat is intercourse? The answers can vary. Some physiologist might equate the workload placed on the body for sexual activity with walking a mile in 20 minutes or climbing 2 flights of stairs in 10 seconds. I would caution doctors viewing sex as purely physical while neglecting the invisible side best described as emotional arousal. Emotional arousal can trigger the release of adrenaline which can have a major impact on blood pressure and pulse.

New sexual encounters or risky sexual impromptu to affairs can raise the heart beat 20 pulse beats or higher than with a regular partner. Men in general like and take risk when it comes to having sex on the run. The new questions should be are you healthy enough to have sex with intense emotional arousal and adrenaline surges? We now know that sexercise can offer one a light to moderate workout. Will it cause a heart attack?

The long awaited answer is a qualified yes. Studies conducted by cardiologist indicate that in the 2 hour period after sex, the risk of having a heart attack increases 2.5 times. The likelihood for most men is still low when you compare the absolute day to day risk taken when we play sports or dance our butt off. Being physically and emotionally fit only further insures our health and wellbeing when it comes to passionate sex. If you want passionate sex or have a playboy lifestyle with women, make sure you maintain peak fitness. For those who play it safe with a customary partner your risk is substantially lower or in the safety zone. When it comes to sex the menu reads light- moderate- or intense. Men should avoid the trying to be super intense all the time. The heart is definitely a strong marker of sexual health. There are still other body markers for good sex that needs to be considered.

Do you have back pains and bad knees?
Well according to Chinese medicine these are symptoms of what is called unbalanced kidney qi (energy). The concept of qi is becoming more common in the west today. Every function of one's body requires sustained energy. There are herbal formulations and special exercises which will be discussed later to help balance the qi levels in the body. Having low back pains and knee problems can really interfere with our ability to have and enjoy sex.

How does blood circulation affect my sex life?

In order to achieve an erection blood must be able to flow to the peripheral area of our bodies such as the penis. If circulation is impaired by any arterial diseases or high blood pressure medication, a man will not be able to achieve or sustain an erection. Exercise in general is one of the best cures for enhancing blood circulation to all areas of the body. Stress on the other hand, can constrict blood vessels and significantly reduce their flow. An all natural vasodilator such as gingko biloba and nervine herb such as passion flower can be very helpful in remedying this problem.

Am I emotionally and mentally balanced?

Sexual activity should be a positive and pleasant experience between two consensual people. Sex can also cause men to experience negative emotions such as disappointment, anxiety, humiliation and frustration and even rage. This can easily happen if men feel that the quality and standards of sex they seek is not possible. Impotency and anguish are often the result. All men should learn to forgive themselves and strive to correct these problems rather than worrying about them.

What are 3 most common diseases that can impairs sex directly or indirectly?

If you guess correctly, they are heart disease, stress, diabetes and hypertension. These diseases can incapacitate a man's performance directly or due to the side effects of medication. These diseases must be kept under proper control while one is seeking a life style change leading to a more permanent cure.

Do you sleep 6-8 hours per night?

Lack of adequate REM sleep can cause many of our hormones to be out of balance. Testosterone and dopamine levels usually rest themselves at night. Many neurotransmitters do not function well when there is sleep deprivation. All the sex pills in the world can not compare to the rejuvenating effect of a good night sleep. Night sleep rebalances and promotes healthy hormone levels especially testosterone.

Our bodies heal itself by regenerating cells and organs restoring us to a more helpful balance. Pushing our bodies beyond our energy reserve will inevitably weaken our bodies triggering our immune system to go into overdrive. Our immune system consumes huge volumes of energy balancing itself daily. Without a good night of sleep one can only expect a lower threshold of energy for sex. Sexual vitality works best when there is a surplus or reserve energy or qi in the body.

Do you drink excessively?

A small amount of alcohol can be beneficial for sex. A small amount of alcohol can actually dilate and relax blood vessels resulting in increase blood flow to the penis and internal organs. In contrast, excessive consumption of alcohol can literally turn off the pilot light of vitality. Even moderate alcohol consumption tends to decrease the vital sex nutrient, zinc. Keep in mind, that zinc is a necessary precursor for the production of testosterone.

Excess alcohol will impair or slow down the necessary vitality and adrenaline we need to have sex. No man wants to go to sleep on the job of making love.

Are you a smoker?

Smoking is definitely out of the question. Smoking is equally bad due to the depletion of oxygen in the body. Lack of oxygen can rob the blood cells of energy and reduce flow to the sex organs. When oxygen levels are reduced to the brain by excess smoking the quality and volume of blood flow to the penis will also diminish. A man's breathing capacity may very well be an index of his potential strength and sexual endurance. Without proper breathing a man can not control his ejaculation or erectile strength. The breath of life must be respected and cultivated. Where there is breath there is life. The more lively a man is the deeper he breathes and the more sexual vitality is at his command.

References:

Marc Perry, CSCS, CPT | February 21, 2012 | Updated: June 4, 2013 JAMA and Archives Journals. "Fitness Level, Not Body Fat, May Be Stronger Predictor Of Longevity For Older Adults." ScienceDaily. ScienceDaily, 5 December 2007. <www.sciencedaily.com/releases/2007/12/071204163249.htm>. Kaptchuk, TedChinese Medicine, The Web That has no Weaver Rider, London, 1983 (Kidney Qi

Mirone V, Ricci E, Gentile V, Basile Fasolo C, Parazzini F. Determinants of erectile dysfunction risk in a large series of Italian men attending andrology clinics. Eur Urol. 2004;45:87–91. [PubMed]

4. The Way of the Herb, Michael Tierra, 1998 Pocket books, Gingko p. 139-140.

5. Van Thiel DH, Lester R. The effect of chronic alcohol abuse on sexual function. th Clin Endocrinol Metab. 1979;8:499–510. [PubMed]

6. Jensen SB, Gludd C. Sexual dysfunction in men with alcoholic liver cirrhosis: A comparative study. Liver.

1985;5:94–100. [PubMed]

7. Mirone V, Ricci E, Gentile V, Basile Fasolo C, Parazzini F. Determinants of erectile dysfunction risk in a large series of Italian men attending andrology clinics. Eur Urol. 2004; 45:87–91. [PubMed]

8. Van Thiel DH, Lester R. The effect of chronic alcohol abuse on sexual function. th Clin Endocrinol Metab. 1979; 8:499–510. [PubMed]

9. Jensen SB, Gludd C. Sexual dysfunction in men with alcoholic liver cirrhosis: A comparative study. Liver. 1985;5:94–100. [PubMed]

10.   Heart Rate, Rate-Pressure Product, and Oxygen Uptake During Four Sexual Activities Joseph G. Bohlen, MD, PhD; James P. Held, BChE; M. Olwen Sanderson, MD; Robert P. Patterson, PhD *Arch   Intern   Med.*   1984;144(9):1745-1748. doi:10.1001/archinte.1984.00350210057007

11. National Institutes of Health, National Heart, Lung, and Blood Institute. *Morbidity & Mortality: 1998 Chartbook on Cardiovascular, Lung and Blood Disease.* U.S. Dept. of Health and Human Services, October, 1998. (Accessed 11/4/99 at http://www.nhlbi.nih.gov/resources/docs/98chtbk.pdf).

12. Ngen, C.C., Quek, D.K., Ong, S.B. Sexual morbidity after myocardial infarction. Med J Malaya. 1991;46:35–40.

13. Papadopoulos, C., Larrimore, P., Cardin, S., Shelley, S.I. Sexual concerns and needs of the postcoronary patient's wife. Arch Intern Med. 1980;140:38–41.

14. Steinke, E., Patterson-Midgley, P. Sexual counseling following acute myocardial infarction. Clin Nurs Res. 1996; 5:462–472.

Chapter 3

The Biology and Chemistry of Libido Simplified

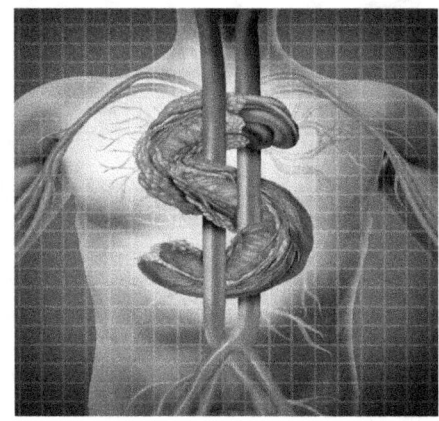

The biology and chemistry of sex is sometimes difficult to fathom for the average non medical layman. There are numerous bio-chemical processes involving enzymes, hormones, vasodilators and neural brain transmitters all working in sync with each other at the right time to make one's libido and sex life work.

Many men often ask why is it necessary to understand these underlying processes in order to have a healthy sex life. The answer is often simple. What you don't know can harm or hinder your potential. In terms of problems related to sex, you can't fix something if you don't know what needs to be fixed. Impotency or lack of sex drive can be symptomatic of many health problems and must be addressed in an individualized manner. The one pill fits all approach certainly does not work for everyone. Viagra or cialis should not be the first step taken when things are not going well in the bedroom most men tend to look for a quick fix rather than a long term solution.

A quick fix will not withstand the test of time nor is it necessarily good for one's health. Men should not opt to jeopardize their overall long term health for the momentary delight of a sexual encounter. I am sure many of us have heard the argument, if I am going to die, then I rather die having sex, as justification to taking steroids, synthetic testosterone and overdosing on sex pills.

Here's a quick test.

What is the most important organ in the body that having good sex depends upon the most? Pause!

The answer is the brain. Sexual arousal starts in the mind by way of perception or anticipation of an erotic event. If your body and mind are not working in harmony, you will not be able to perform as you desire.

Engaging in a sexual act requires mental focus as well as physical energy.

Let us begin our lesson with defining a few simple terms such as hormone, enzyme, vasodilator and a brain neurotransmitter.

Hormones are biochemical messengers that are released from glands in the body to trigger specific physical processes such as the release testosterone, adrenaline and estrogen to name a few. They also tend to bind to receptor sites in the body where they are needed.

Enzymes are biochemical compounds that speed up or enable certain reactions to occur. An example of this would be aromatase which triggers the unfortunate conversion of free flowing testosterone into estrogen. Vasodilators refer to a class of substances that can expand or open up a blood vessel and increase its flow. Aspirin is a common example.

Brain neurotransmitters are brain chemicals like hormones that can turn on or off specific reactions in the body. A good example of this compound is the euphoric blissful bonding experienced following an orgasm due to the release of oxytocin and endorphins. The love hormone, oxytocin is known to be plentiful in lactating women and is released by both men and women after an orgasm.

What causes an erection?

Erection of the penis is one of the most important physiological processes to occur in males regardless of their age, genetic make-up or geographic location. Most men usually associate the erection of the penis with sexual arousal. This is not necessary true. Erections can occur on a regular basis without the premeditated thought of a sexual arousing image or event. The average healthy male can have 4-8 erections at night while sleeping and dreaming. There are 3 distinct stages of penile erection.

Arousal: The man becomes sexually aroused via thought and association.

Erection: The penis responds by becoming erect and firm.

Ejaculation: Physical stimulation of the penis causes the release of semen. If, by any chance, step two (erection) does not happen, step three (ejaculation) becomes difficult or almost impossible. This condition can lead to what is called "male impotence".

What is the role of the brain in causing an erection?

The penis is one of the places in the body where the brain needs to be able to turn the blood flow on and off with a thought. When a man is sexually stimulated by sight, thought, or touch, the brain sends signals that relax the smooth muscles around the arteries that supply blood to the corpora cavernosa. The veins draining the blood cannot keep up, resulting in swelling. As the swelling reaches the limit of the penile skin, the penis becomes firm.

The pressure of the spongy corpora cavernosa against the skin partially closes the veins, helping to maintain the erection. Erection continues until the signals from the brain stop, but erections are seldom consistent. Waxing and waning like the moon are normal responses even during intercourse.

What is the role of the corpora cavernosa?

The penis uses a similar mechanism, but instead of using pressurized air to become rigid, the penis uses pressurized blood. The penis contains two cigar-shaped structures, called corpora cavernosa (singular: corpus cavernosum), that it uses to become erect. You can think of the corpora cavernosa as balloon-like tubes. Arteries bring blood into these two tubes and veins carry blood away from them.

The penis can be either limp or erect, depending on the flow of blood. Inside the shaft of the penis are three columns of erectile tissue—the two corpora cavernosa, which run parallel to each other along the top of the penis, and the corpus spongiosum, which runs along the bottom of the penis and surrounds the urethra.

Despite the fact that erections are often called "boners," there are no bones within the penis. During an erection, the corpora cavernosa and the corpus spongiosum, which are rich in blood vessels become engorged with blood. This expansion makes the penis larger and firmer. The fancy name for this is "vaso-congestion." In a non-erect state, the arteries that bring blood into the corpora cavernosa are somewhat constricted, while the veins that drain the blood from the penis are open. There is no way for pressure to build inside the penis. In this state, the penis is limp. When a man becomes aroused, the arteries leading into the penis open up so that pressurized blood can enter the penis quickly.

The veins leaving the penis constrict. Pressurized blood is trapped in the corpora cavernosa, and this blood causes the penis to elongate and stiffen. The penis is now erect. If the arteries leading to the penis do not open up properly, it is difficult or impossible for a man to become erect.

This problem is the leading cause of erectile dysfunction (ED). To solve an erection problem when the cause is poor blood flow, you need to open the arteries. There are natural safe non invasive methods to achieve this goal. I will discuss these methods later. In addition to producing sperm, the testicles also produce male hormones, including testosterone. Testosterone has a sizable effect on sexual desire, and, in turn, sexual desire is often the first stage in sexual arousal and erection. If the testicles are removed and testosterone production slows or stops, then sexual desire typically decreases, and erections may be fewer or nonexistent.

The prostate is a gland that surrounds the urethra in men and produces about 30% of the fluid that makes up what is called ejaculate or "cum." It is also a gland that is particularly prone to cancer, especially as men age. It is important to get regular prostate examinations if you are 50 years or older. Treatments for prostate cancer, including surgical removal of the prostate, can cause erectile dysfunction (an inability to get an erection). This is not because the prostate is necessary to have an erection, but most likely because of the nerve or blood vessel damage caused by surgery or radiation treatments. Psychological trauma can also result from prostate removal. It can be said more often, take care of your prostate if you still have one.

What are some of the most common causes of ED or impotency in males?

As you might expect there are numerous medical conditions that can render a healthy sexual warrior inert. Behind the scenes, a lot goes into achieving an erection. When you're turned on, nerves fire in your brain and travel down your spinal cord to your penis. There, muscles relax and blood flows into the blood vessels. If all goes well, a firm penis is now ready for sex. Unfortunately, all does not always go well. Many diseases their treatment can lead to erectile dysfunction (ED). Injuries, lifestyle choices, and other physical factors are known to play a significant role. ED can often be treated, and finding the right cause can lead to successful treatment.

Diabetes: This chronic disease can damage the nerves and blood vessels that aid in getting an erection. When the disease has not been well controlled over time, it can double a man's risk of erection problems.

Kidney Disease: Kidney disease can affect many of the things you need for a healthy erection, including your hormones, blood flow to your penis, and parts of your nervous system. It can also sap your energy level and rob you of your sex drive. Drugs for kidney disease can also cause ED.

Neurological Disorders: You can't get an erection without help from your nervous system. Diseases that disrupt signals between your brain and your penis can lead to ED. Such diseases include stroke, multiple sclerosis (MS), alzheimer's disease, and parkinson's disease.

Blood Vessel Diseases: Vascular diseases can block the blood vessels. That slows the flow of blood to the penis, making an erection difficult to get. Atherosclerosis (hardening of the arteries), high blood pressure, and high cholesterol are among the most common causes of ED.

Prostate Cancer: Prostate cancer doesn't cause ED, but treatments can lead to temporary or permanent erectile dysfunction.
The physical causes of ED are not only just disease-related. There are many other potential causes such as
surgery. Surgery for both prostate cancer and bladder
cancer can damage nerves and tissues necessary for an erection. Sometimes the problem may clear up within 6 to 18 months or the damage can be more permanent. If that happens, treatments are available to help restore a man's ability to have an erection.

Injury: Injuries to the pelvis, bladder, spinal cord, and penis that require surgery also can cause ED.

Hormone Problems: Testosterone and other hormones fuel a man's sex drive. An imbalance can throw off his interest in sex. Dopamine, an important brain neurotransmitter can influence testosterone levels and sex drive via mood when being aroused. If dopamine levels are too low the craving and urge for sex are diminished. Causes can include pituitary gland tumors, kidney and liver disease, depression, and hormone treatment of prostate cancer.

Venous Leak: To keep an erection, the blood that flows into your penis must stay in your penis. If it flows back out too quickly a condition called venous leak can occur. When the veins in your penis don't constrict properly you will lose your erection. Both injuries and disease can cause venous leak.

Tobacco, Alcohol, or Drugs: All three can damage your blood vessels. That makes it difficult for blood to reach the penis, which is essential for an erection. If you have hardened arteries (arteriosclerosis), smoking will dramatically raise your risk of ED.

Prescription Drugs: There are more than 200 prescription drugs that can cause ED as a result of their side effects.

Prostate Enlargement: Prostate enlargement, a normal part of aging for many men, may also play a role in ED.

We can clearly see that the enemy can come from within and without. The sexual warrior must be aware of the disabling or crippling power of these medical conditions and strive to avoid or prevent them. One must never give up hope to cure or mitigate these conditions. There are also emotional or psychological issues that can be just as devastating as the medical problems.

Erectile Dysfunction can also be caused by emotional problems:

Worry

Fear

Stress

Anger

Depression

Lack of interest in sex, or in the sexual partner

Good or Bad Testosterone

All forms of testosterone are not the same. A good comparison to testosterone is cholesterol.

Most people are keenly aware that cholesterol can be good or bad. The bad cholesterol is called LDL. The good cholesterol is called HDL. Most doctors prefer there patients have a higher ratio of HDL to LDL to help prevent heart disease. Cholesterol in itself is a very beneficial substance to the body. Most of our hormones are actually made from cholesterol. The normal to healthy range is 130 -200 for total cholesterol profile. What is considered to be the normal range is disputable. Many life and health insurance companies cholesterol reference range for acceptability is 200-300. A cholesterol of 245 may be optimal if the ratio of LDL to HDL is good. Higher HDL levels tend to neutralize the bad LDL.

Other Intrinsic Factors

1. Pelvic floor structure and function are also positively influenced by sexual activity and can lead to positive feedback mechanisms by increasing pleasurable feeling. There is at the same time also a preventive effect on the development of prolapse and incontinence.

2. The endocrine changes especially related to orgasm include oxytocin and dopamine secretions, and may thus change the internal neuroendocrine milieu involved in general affective states. This may even reduce the risk of depression.

3. The emotional reactions include body-related feelings of excitement, pleasure, and relaxation, which in a medium- and long-term perspective may have a positive impact on body image and internal body representation, thus preventing body image disorders and functional somatic syndromes.

REFERENCES

1. Krieger L. Scoring before a big event. Winning 1997; 1:88–89.

2. Bloom M. The sex factor. Runner's World 1994; 11:71–74.

3. Johnson W. Muscular performance following coitus. J Sex Res 1968; 4:247–248.

4. Thornton J. Sexual activity and athletic performance: is there a relationship? Phys Sport Med 1990; 18:148–153.

5. Boone T, Gilmore S. Effects of sexual intercourse on maximal aerobic power, oxygen pulse, and double product in male sedentary subjects. J Sports Med Phys Fitness 1995; 35:214–217.

6. Mirkin G. Sex before competition. Report #6750. Mar. 10, 1996. http://drmirkin.com/archive/6750.html

7. Anshel M. Effects of sexual activity on athletic performance. Phys Sports Med 1981; 9:65–68.

8. Bohlen J, Held J, Sanderson M, et al. Heart rate, rate pressure point, and oxygen uptake during four sexual activities. Arch Intern Med 1984; 144:1745–1748.

9. Clinical Journal of Sport Medicine:
October 2000 - Volume 10 - Issue 4 - pp 233-234

Chapter 4

Can Sex Make You Healthy?

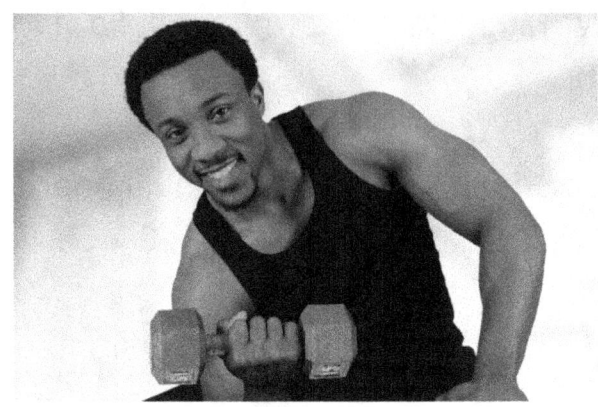

In the previous chapters we discussed how to determine if a person is healthy enough to engage in sexual activity. Sometimes the idea of having sex is a lot easier to conceive than the act itself. It makes sense that just having the urge for sex or feeling horny can a good sign of heightened libido or testosterone. In other words, if you desire or crave to have sex, the ability to do so is usually intact, such as adequate dopamine levels. Can sex make you healthy? The answer to this question has at least two sides or perspectives in being able to solve or come up with a solution. If sex can make you healthy then it stands to reason that sex can also make you sick as well.

Our brains play a key role when it comes to having healthy sex. Proper activation of the hypothalamic–pituitary–testicular axis is of paramount importance in jump starting your sex life. Increased T levels, shorter recovery between sexual activity and readiness for follow up sexual encounters are all positive signs for sexual health.

Sex is Important for Both the Body as Well as The Mind.

Most people just don't view sex and love making as a way to strengthen their muscles, tendons, ligaments and internal organs. Most don't think of it as a way to keep you younger, improve your circulation and enhance your performance for sports. Strengthening your sex muscle can make you more creative and can attract success in your life.

The other side the coin deal with the question, "are you healthy enough to have sex or can sex make you healthy?" Many sex researchers believe that healthy sex can make men and women look up to 7 years younger than their peer counterpart. There are many explanations why this may be true. Regular sex tends to trigger the release of endorphins which acts as a natural pain killer and stress reduction modifier. Less anxiety and stress helps to improve our quality of sleep. Sex in itself is a form of exercise that stimulates circulation and improves heart heath. The release of human growth hormones while engaging in sex can make the skin look more elastic.

One research study found that people who looked younger than their age had sex 50 percent more often than people of similar age. The study found that people who looked younger in their 40s and 50s had sex on average three times per week compared to "older looking" people who had sex just twice a week. Sexual satisfaction is an important contributor to the quality of one's life. Having sex may even rank as high as spiritual or religious commitment and other morale factors. Everyone should try to attain a more positive attitude towards sex. Being sexually active is a prerogative for both mature young and older people. There are more reasons to have sex than to restrict oneself from it. Not only can sex make you feel good but it can also make you smarter.

Human beings by nature have a powerful sex drive and strive to learn how to control and harness this sexual energy. Men should be aware of these sexual practices in order to develop longevity, power, and physical strength. The hormones and nutrients of sexual activity create new life. These internal nutrients can be recycled to make our lives longer and more enjoyable. Over 2000 years ago only the Chinese emperors, his consorts and the emperors' advisors like the shaolin monks.

With deeper knowledge and understanding you'll make love consciously and with a totally different intention. The emotional power of sex can be quite exhilarating. Although this lost art of lovemaking comes from China, it was kept hidden from the masses or common people. Even to this day, the practices are still well guarded. For the most part, the only people who knew it were royalty, imperial consorts, shaolin and taoist monks. Miraculously, these people are the ones who live the longest, look the best, and appear to attract success like magic. The emotional power of sex properly harnessed can be used to accomplish anything and everything you want out of life!

6 Key Benefits for Having Sex

1. Boost Brain Power

As mentioned above, yes, sex can make you smarter! In fact, according to a new research study in Maryland and South Korea, (Hippocampus. 2013 Apr;23(4):303-12. doi: 10.1002/hipo.22090. Epub 2013 Mar 5.

2. **The R**estoration of Age-Related Mental Decline

Sex can improve one's mental performance and it helps produce more new neurons in the hippocampus, where long-term memories are formed. Researchers from the University of Maryland have performed several experiments on middle-aged rats to prove it. What they've found is that when these rats were allowed to have sex, they showed signs of more improved cognitive and hippocampus function.

3. **Stress Buster and Lowers High Blood Pressure**

It is a known fact that sex can dilate blood vessels due to the increased presence of nitric oxide. Also, people who engage in sexual activity at least twice a week are observed to be happier and less stressed.

4. Headache and Pain Reliever

In the March issue of the Journal Cephalagia, it was found that sex can relieve headache pains. Patients who have used sex as a therapy to cure their migraines or headaches can do so without the risk of over medication.

5. Immune System Booster

Research has already shown that sex can help boost your immune system. In fact, it says that it can even help you prevent getting the flu. This is because during sexual activity higher levels of immunoglobulins (IMGS) are produced. The IMGS which is an antibody can prevent colds and flus when you have sex at least 2-3times a week. Researchers have seen good immune responses from people who had sex at least 2 times per week. When compared to people who had no sex, those who had sex at least twice a week got a much better immune response.

6. Sleep Aid

Sex can improve your sleep. If you are suffering from sleep deprivation or having difficulty sleeping and you don't want to take medications, then you may want to engage in a sexual activity more often.

Competition and Sport Performance

The long-standing myth that athletes should practice abstinence before important competitions may stem from the theory that sexual frustration leads to increased aggression. The act of ejaculation can draw testosterone from the body. In a study done with 14 married male former athletes, they were given a maximum-effort grip strength test the morning after intercourse. The same test was given after 6 days of abstinence.

The results suggested that strength and endurance of the palmar flexing muscles are not adversely affected by sex the previous night. An unpublished follow-up to this study was conducted by researchers at Colorado State University on 10 fit, married men, ages 18–45 years. In their tests for grip strength, balance, lateral movement, reaction time, aerobic power (stair-climbing exercise), and VO_{2max} (treadmill test), the results did not change with sexual activity. Finally, the results from a 1995 randomized cross-over study suggested that sexual intercourse 12 hours prior to the test had no significant effects on maximal aerobic power, oxygen pulse, or double product. Considering that normal sexual intercourse between married partners expends only 25–50 calories (the energy equivalent of walking up two flights of stairs), it is doubtful that sex the previous night would affect laboratory physiological performance tests.

Prior to any athletic event a small degree of anxiety can be good to make the athlete more alert and ready to explode in the event. Being too anxious or not alert enough can hinder performance at any time. If athletes are too anxious and restless the night before an event, then sex may be a relaxing distraction. Some athletes have little interest in sex the night before a big competition. This theory predicts that the results will be dependent on individual preferences and routines. The night before an important race is not a good time for drastic changes in routine. Consistency is the key.

As legendary New York Yankees manager Casey Stengel put it, "It's not the sex that wrecks these guys, it's staying up all night looking for it." The long-standing myth that athletes should practice abstinence before important competitions may stem from the theory that sexual frustration leads to increased aggression, and that the act of ejaculation draws testosterone from the body. How this extra boost in testosterone is used depends partially upon the athletes conditioning program and mental focus. Added adrenaline rush can also negatively impact an athlete causing him to try to hard to win while sacrificing mental strategy and flexibility.

REFERENCES:

1. Krieger L. Scoring before a big event. Winning 1997; 1:88–89.

2. Bloom M. The sex factor. Runner's World 1994; 11:71–74.

3. Johnson W. Muscular performance following coitus. J Sex Res 1968; 4:247–248.

4. Thornton J. Sexual activity and athletic performance: is there a relationship? Phys Sport Med 1990; 18:148–153.

5. Boone T, Gilmore S. Effects of sexual intercourse on maximal aerobic power, oxygen pulse, and double product in male sedentary subjects. J Sports Med Phys Fitness 1995; 35:214–217.

6. Mirkin G. Sex before competition. Report #6750. Mar. 10, 1996. http://drmirkin.com/archive/6750.html

7. Anshel M. Effects of sexual activity on athletic performance. Phys Sports Med 1981; 9:65–68.

8. Bohlen J, Held J, Sanderson M, et al. Heart rate, rate pressure point, and oxygen uptake during four sexual activities. Arch Intern Med 1984; 144:1745–1748.

9. Graham JM, Desjardins C. Classical conditioning: Induction of luteinizing hormone and testosterone secretion in anticipation of sexual activity. Science 1980;210:1039–41.

10 Fox CA, Ismail AA, Love DN, Kirkham KE, Loraine JA. Studies on the relationship between

plasma testosterone levels and human sexual activity. J Endocrinol 1972;52:51–8.

11 Hirschenhauser K, Frigerio D, Grammer K, Magnusson MS. Monthly patterns of testosterone and behavior in prospective fathers. Horm Behav 2002;42:172–81.

13, DiMeo PJ. Psychosocial and relationship issues in men with erectile dysfunction. Urol Nurs. 2006 Dec;26(6):442-6, 453; quiz 447.

14. Tikkanen MJ, Jackson G, Tammela T, et al. Erectile dysfunction as a risk factor for coronary heart disease: implications for prevention. Int J Clin Pract. 2007 Feb;61(2):265-8.

15.   Booth A, Johnson DR, Granger DA. Testosterone and men's health. J Behav Med. 1999; 22:1-19

16.   Clinical Journal of Sport Medicine:
October 2000 - Volume 10 - Issue 4 - pp 233-234
Editoria

Chapter 5

The Testosterone Connection

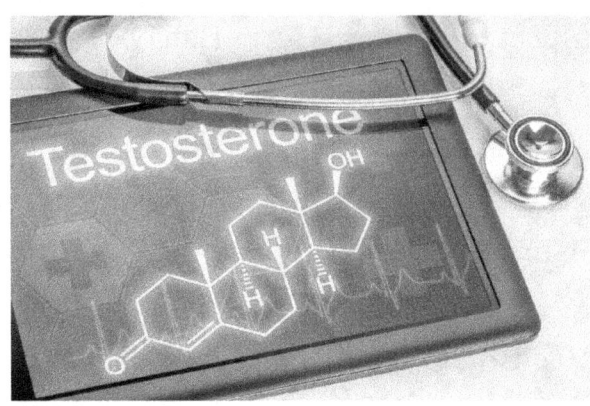

When examining the major bio-markers for male health the androgen hormone testosterone could easily take first place. What is exactly testosterone and why is it so important? Testosterone belongs to a group of hormones called *androgens* also referred to as male hormones. Testosterone is the hormone responsible for the growth and development of male genetalia as well as male sex characteristics such as chest, facial and pubic hair, vocal characteristics, and muscle growth.

How is the testosterone connection being threatened today for most men?

1. Genetically modified foods and toxins in our water can deplete testosterone production for the average male.

2. Studies show men with low testosterone levels have a 74% higher death rate than those with normal levels.

3. Men can lose up to 90% of their testosterone between the ages of 25 and 90 years old.

4.   Cellular telephone and other wi-fi devices radiation exposure of 60 minutes or more can deplete testosterone. Keep your cell phone out of your pants pocket.

In Chinese terms, both the yin and yang need to be balanced. If your hormone and testosterone levels have declined then you're probably waking up "tired and sexually depleted" more often than you'd like to admit. When out of balance, men become more Yin - or feminine.

A deficiency of testosterone can manifest as these symptoms:

- Low sex drive (libido)
- Erectile dysfunction
- Fatigue and low energy levels
- Difficulty concentrating
- Depression
- Irritability
- Low sense of well-being

Potential Benefits From Increased Testosterone Levels Include:

- Increase in lean body mass
- Decreased levels of triglycerides and LDL cholesterol (bad cholesterol)
- Increase libido and improved sexual performance
- Improvement in insulin sensitivity & reduced risk of type-2 diabetes
- Increased energy and stamina
- Improved circulatory system health
- Reduced estradiol production
- Decreased risk of osteoporosis
- Reduction in risk of cardio-vascular disease
- Boosts anabolic hormone levels

Liver Health

Are you healthy enough for sex also depends upon the condition of your liver. The liver is one of the few internal organs that can regenerate itself like the tail of a gecko lizard when it is cut off as long as the liver remains in good condition. Many men tend to drink more alcohol than can be safely processed by the liver. Overtime the liver can become congested and hardened leading to a condition known as sclerosis pf the liver. Many fail to appreciate the important role of the liver as it relates to health and sex.

Having a healthy functioning liver is definitely a prerequisite for healthy sex. The liver does all sorts of wonderful things in our lives. It metabolizes human growth hormones (HGH) into IGF-2 and filters the blood from toxins. Part of the liver function is to release a protein called the sex binding globulin or SHBG in order to regulate the level of testosterone from being too high. Sometimes the liver does its job too well producing more SHBG than needed. The result of this action by the liver can cause testosterone to be bounded and carried away before the body has a chance to use it. Bounded testosterone has no bioavailability. It tends to float around in the bloodstream while attached to a protein unable to interact with any receptors in the body. SHBG now becomes junk and have to be removed by the liver.

Since we cannot live very long without a liver due to its key functions, its best to leave this organ alone and treat the SHBG in the bloodstream instead. Any alteration of the liver function can have a negative domino effect on the rest of the body. One of the most effective means of neutralizing SHBG comes not from the pharmacy but rather the roots of a common weed. This weed is known as stinging nettle.

Testosterone testing can measure the level of this male hormone (androgen) in the blood. Testosterone affects sexual features and development. In men, it is made in large amounts by the testicles. In both men and women, testosterone is made in small amounts by the adrenal glands, and in women, by the ovaries. The controlling factor for the production of testosterone is the pituitary gland.

The pituitary gland controls the level of testosterone in the body. When the testosterone level is low, the pituitary gland releases a hormone called luteinizing hormone (LH). This hormone signals a man's testicles to make more testosterone. Before puberty, the testosterone level in boys is normally low. Testosterone increases during puberty. This causes boys to develop a deeper voice, get bigger muscles, make sperm, and develop facial and body hair. The level of testosterone is highest around age 40, it gradually becomes less in older men. The difference between men under 40 is the amount of conversion of testosterone to estrogen and free available testosterone in their blood. Younger men tend to have more free available unbound testosterone circulating hormones than older ones. Most of the testosterone produced by older men is converted by enzymes such as aromatase into estrogenic compounds.

Most of the testosterone in the blood is bound to the sex hormone binding globulin (SHBG). Testosterone that is not bound or free testosterone may be checked if a man or a woman is having sexual problems. Free testosterone also may be tested for a person who has a condition that can change SHBG levels, such as hyperthyroidism or some types of kidney diseases. Total testosterone levels vary throughout the day. They are usually highest in the morning and lowest in the evening.

Healthy men young and old tend to have less fat receptors and more lean muscles to resist the absorption of estrogen. Being over weight, having long-term (chronic) pain, or taking pain medicines can lower the level of sex hormone. This also decreases total testosterone level. If a man's body fat composition is high, he will attract more estrogen molecules into his body tissues. In women, the ovaries account for half of the testosterone in the body. Women have a much smaller amount of testosterone in their bodies compared to men. But testosterone plays an important role throughout the body in both men and women. It affects the brain, bone and muscle mass, fat distribution, the vascular system, energy levels, genital tissues, and sexual functioning.

Here is a reference chart on the normal range for testosterone

Total Testosterone [1]	
Men	270–1070 ng/Dl (9–38 nmo/L)
Women	15–70 ng/dL (0.52–2.4 nmol/L)
Children (depends on sex and age at puberty)	2–20 ng/dL or 0.07–0.7 nmol/L

Free Testosterone Reference Range [1]	
Men	50–210 pg/mL (174–729 pmol/L)
Women	1.0–8.5 pg/mL (3.5–29.5 pmol/L)

Free testosterone only makes up about 2% of the body's total testosterone profile. It is however the most important component that defines a man's masculine traits. Putting this into perspective should help men realize that it's all about quality of testosterone present rather than quantity.

Luteinizing hormones, may be checked to see whether a low testosterone level is caused by problems with the testicles or ovaries or the pituitary gland. A really high level of LH and a low level of testosterone often means that the testicles or ovaries are not working properly. A low LH level and a really low or high testosterone level may mean a problem with the pituitary gland.

When we examine testosterone, we can easily find similar comparisons to cholesterol. Despite all the warning about the deleterious effect of cholesterol in terms of arterial disease, cholesterol is very important when it comes to good sex. It is cholesterol that makes sex hormones like testosterone. Low levels cholesterol can also indicate low levels of testosterone. The healthy range of cholesterol for the medical community is 150-200. Interestingly enough, the acceptable range in the life insurance industry to qualify clients as healthy and of low risk for heart disease is 200-300.

Why is there not a consensus? The answer lies within the hidden understanding and emphasis placed upon the specific type of cholesterol. It is the ratio of LDL or bad cholesterol to good cholesterol such as HDL that is most important. A cholesterol level of 245 is ideal for the production of testosterone for sex and body building if the ratio of HDL is higher than the LDL level. It is the HDL levels that prevent heart disease and protects the arteries from plaque. This is the reason why insurance companies have set their reference range for healthy cholesterol higher than the medical community. The medical community tends to favor the use of medication to control cholesterol creating a fear base atmosphere to promote the sale of drugs like statin.

Testosterone can come in several forms, the good, bad and most beneficial. The sometimes bad testosterone is called (DHT), which stands for dihydrotestosterone. DHT can sometimes cause prostates to swell and male pattern baldness if in excess. The good form is your total testosterone level index. The most beneficial form is what is referred to as the free unbound testosterone which constitutes only 2% of the total testosterone produced by a healthy male. It is the free unbounded testosterone that gives men stronger sex drives, harder erections and more masculine physical traits.

Prostate Health

Are you healthy enough for sex depends upon the condition of the prostate gland. The formation of DHT or the unhealthy testosterone can cause the prostate to enlarge due to its effect on the prostate cells. This condition can lead to what is called benign prostatic hypertrophy or enlarged prostate, BPH. A swollen prostate is not conducive for healthy sex. BPH can cause frequent trips to the bathroom, erection problems and at worst set up the growth of cancer cells.

It is the body's rogue enzyme 5 alpha reductase that converts testosterone into DHT in prostate tissue. I highly recommend the use of cruciferous vegetables, herbs like stinging nettle and saw palmetto to improve male potency, increase fertility, reduce inflammation and swelling of the prostate gland. These herbs not only provide the necessary nutrition for a healthy prostate but also strengthen other glands in the body. Saw Palmetto is the best-known for its affect on sexual function.

Today more than ever, we see a commercial explosion in the use of medical testosterone and anabolic steroids products. The availability of these products may not be a good thing. Testosterone replacement therapy is only appropriate and safe for men who have below-normal levels and who don't have any medical conditions that could be made worse by testosterone. This includes conditions such as an enlarged prostate or evidence of prostate cancer. The use of testosterone by men with normal levels is very risky. The symptoms of hypogonadism or shrunken balls are often overlooked, because they are often mistaken for ordinary signs of aging.

The enormous industry that has sprung up to capitalize on this problem has contributed to a dangerous rise in the unregulated sale and use of testosterone supplements. Far too many men are accessing quick-and unhealthy prescriptions for testosterone because it makes them feel temporarily younger and stronger.

Myth Buster 1

Men can raise their testosterone levels by exercising vigorously.

The relationship between testosterone and exercise is complicated. Yes, moderate exercise can raise testosterone levels to a limited extent. If however, exercises are extreme, testosterone levels can actually drop. There is a point of diminishing returns due to over training. It's also true that low testosterone can make it harder to exercise consistently which can lead to a vicious cycle of inactivity and reduced hormone levels.

Myth Buster 2

Erection-enhancing medications (such as Viagra) work whether a man has normal testosterone levels or not.

Studies show that erection-enhancing medications work best in men with testosterone levels in the normal range. Testosterone provides the necessary urge or libido desire to initiate sex that erection-enhancing drugs cannot provide. The thrill of sex must be present before the act.

Free Report Available on Request
"Sex Herbs , Closely Guarded Secrets Revealed"
Available on request by visiting www.lifeishealing.com

References:

1. RefeFischbach FT, Dunning MB III, eds. (2009). Manual of Laboratory and Diagnostic Tests, 8th ed. Philadelphia: Lippincott Williams and Wilkins.

Other Works Consulted

- Chernecky CC, Berger BJ (2008). Laboratory Tests and Diagnostic Procedures, 5th ed. St. Louis: Saunders.
- Fischbach FT, Dunning MB III, eds. (2009). Manual of Laboratory and Diagnostic Tests, 8th ed. Philadelphia: Lippincott Williams and Wilkins.
- Pagana KD, Pagana TJ (2010). Mosby's Manual of Diagnostic and Laboratory Tests, 4th ed. St. Louis: Mosby Elsevier.

Effects of mobile phone radiation on serum testosterone in Wistar albino rats.

Meo SA, Al-Drees AM, Husain S, Khan MM, Imran MB.
2010 Aug;31(8):869-73.

Low serum testosterone and mortality in male veterans.

Shores MM, Matsumoto AM, Sloan KL, Kivlahan DR.
2006 Aug 14-28;166(15):1660-5.

Chapter 6

The Nitric Oxide Wonder

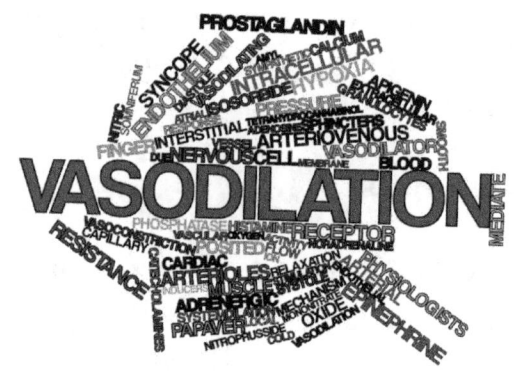

What It Is and How It Works?

Nitric Oxide (NO) is a gas that's naturally produced in the body. The human body makes nitric oxide using enzymes to break down the amino acid known as arginine (often called L-arginine). It's used to communicate messages back and forth between cells. It also plays a key role in controlling the circulation of blood and regulating activities of major organs like the brain, lungs, liver, kidneys, stomach and more. Nitric Oxide also affects the release of hormones and adrenaline, mental focus and a feeling of sharpness.

Nitric oxide is produced by three main enzymes called nitric oxide synthase (NOS). The NOS that has to do with erectile dysfunction is found in the endothelial cells of blood vessels in the penis. This enzyme breaks down l-arginine to create N-O, nitric oxide, which stimulates the cells to produce cyclic GMP or guanosine monophosphate. GMP regulates the movement of ions while signaling the smooth muscle in the blood vessels to relax. Phosphodiesterases, or PDE (sometimes called PDE-5), degrade the GMP, which causes the blood vessels to constrict. PDE-5 is most concentrated in the lungs and penis. There are numerous other substances on the market that can address erectile dysfunction besides drugs.

Nitric Oxide Benefits Can Include

- Increased strength and endurance
- Increased fat loss (in combination with a sensible diet)
- Quicker recovery after physical exertion
- Increased muscle growth
- Increased focus and alertness
- Enhanced libido and may aid erectile dysfunction
- May help reduce pain of joint inflammation and osteoarthritis
- Supports immune system function

Nitric Oxide is neither a mineral nor a vitamin. It is a biological gas that is produced within the body and assists in a variety of physiological functions. It is useful in treating a variety of conditions such as insomnia, obesity, diabetes and sexual problems. It is because of these abilities that NO is touted to be the next miracle cure on the shelf.

Benefits of Nitric Oxide – A Closer Look

- **Blood Circulation** – Nitric Oxide regulates blood circulation throughout the body, increases the diameter of blood vessels and prevents formation of clots. It assists the endothelial cells in controlling and relaxing blood vessels. Nitric Oxide supplementation can increase the oxygen levels within your body, reduce blood pressure levels and keep your heart healthy and functioning optimally.

• **Endurance level** – Nitric Oxide increases the endurance level of the muscle cells, enabling you to lift heavier loads and perform strenuous activities with ease. This is again one of the major reasons why body builders consider nitric oxide supplementation extremely beneficial.

• **Increases Alertness** – Nitric Oxide acts as an intracellular messenger between various cells in the body, including the nerve cells. With adequate amount of NO present in the body, the communication between nerve cells is faster, leading to quick responses and an increase in focus and vigilance.

• **Increases Sexual Energy** – One of the most popular benefits of nitric oxide is that it stimulates, invigorates and amplifies the sexual response mechanism within the body. Sensory and mental stimulation causes the nerve cells to release nitric oxide. This causes the penis muscles to relax, allowing blood to flow into the penis and create an erection. The process remains the same for women too, as blood flow increases in their vaginal tissues. This is how the loss of libido, lack of sexual energy etc can be easily treated with nitric oxide supplementation.

• **Pain Relief**– Nitric Oxide supplementation can provide long-term relief from the pain associated with arthritis and joint inflammation. This is because it activates the anti-inflammatory mechanism within the body cells, and helps in reducing inflammation.

- **Increases Muscle Mass** – Nitric Oxide supplements widen the blood channels that lead to skeletal muscles, allowing for better blood flow and an increase in the lean muscle mass. With an increase in blood flow, the amount of nutrients available for the muscles is more, which again contributes toward increasing their size.

- **Better Intra-cellular Communication** – Nitric Oxide improves the process of communication between various cells in the body, including the nerve and the brain cells. Nitric Oxide supplementation is therefore extremely beneficial for enhancing memory, learning abilities and concentration levels. It also aids in treating various disorders especially insomnia and gastrointestinal ailments.

- **Immune System** – The Immune cells within our body release nitric oxide to destroy bacteria, virus and other harmful foreign elements that can cause an infection. The quality of blood cells in the bone marrow, the immunity-boosting cells and the muscle cells is enhanced with nitric oxide supplements. NO is also known to prevent tumor and cancerous growths within the body cells.

Nitric Oxide supplementation can help everyone, but it is especially beneficial for people over the age of 40. The reason behind this is simple: when you are young, your muscles, body cells and tissues are also in their prime – quick and efficient at releasing and producing enough nitric oxide to carry out different bodily processes.

In addition to all of these benefits, nitric oxide is also a rich source of essential nutrients such as B-sitosterol, ursolic, ghycosides, plant sterols and anthrquinoidenes. It is also rich in zinc, calcium, potassium, iron and vitamin A and C.

Be careful about the dosage – Nitric Oxide supplements contain amino acids which if taken in excess, can lead to diarrhea, nausea and fatigue. With that caveat issued, it is safe to say that NO oxide can help you in more ways than you can think of. As you grow old, your muscles become weaker and the response mechanism of your nerve cells also drops. It is then that you need nitric oxide supplements to boost your cellular activity, increase muscle mass, enhance strength and stamina, and improve your sexual performance. Whatever health problems you may be suffering from – neural, immune system related or gastrointestinal, there is a good chance that nitric oxide supplementation can help you.

Nitric Oxide Conversion Diagram

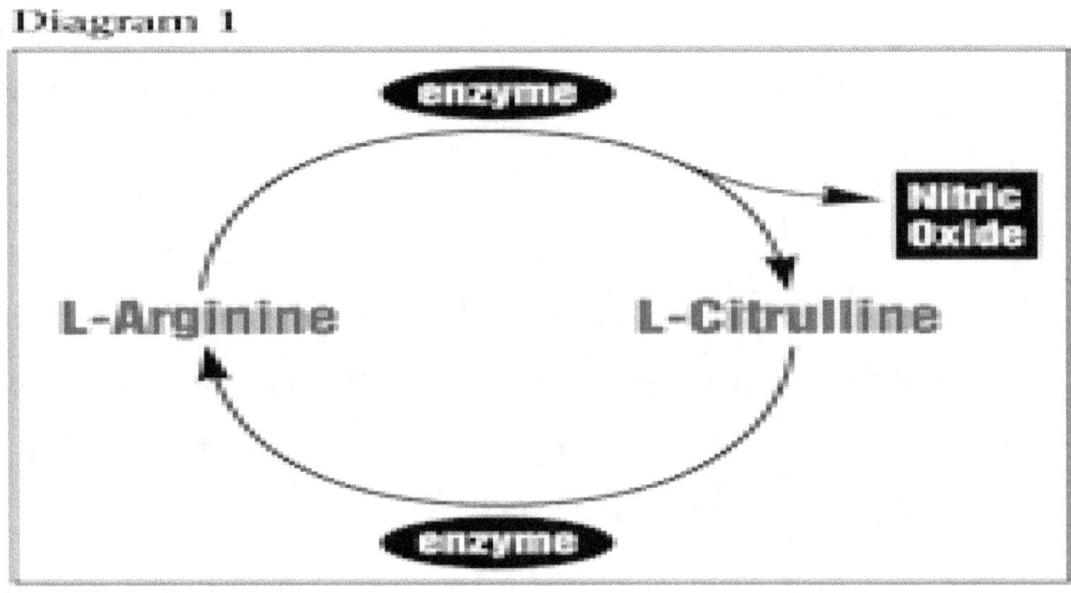

How to Increase Nitric Oxide in Your Body

The most common way to increase nitric oxide is through exercise. When you run or lift weights, your muscles need more oxygen which is supplied by the blood. As the heart pumps with more pressure to supply the muscles with blood, the lining in your arteries releases nitric oxide into the blood. This action relaxes and widens the vessel wall, allowing for more blood to pass though.

As we age, our blood vessels and nitric oxide system become less efficient due to free radical damage, inactivity, and poor diet causing our veins and arteries to deteriorate. Think of a fire hose as water rushes through it to put out a fire. The hose needs to expand enough to handle the pressure, while maintaining enough force to put out the fire. Athletes and youth have the most optimal nitric oxide systems, reflecting their energy and resilience.

Another way to increase nitric oxide is through diet, most notably by consuming the amino acids L-arginine and L-citrulline. Arginine, which can be found in nuts, fruits, dark chocolate, meats and dairy, creates nitric oxide and citrulline inside the cell (see diagram 1). Citrulline is then recycled back into arginine, making even more nitric oxide. Enzymes that convert arginine to citrulline, and citrulline to arginine need to function optimally for efficient nitric oxide production.

We can protect those enzymes and nitric oxide by consuming healthy foods and antioxidants, like fruit, garlic, soy, vitamins C and E, Co-Q10 and alpha lipoic acid which allows you to produce more nitric oxide. Nitric oxide only lasts a few seconds in the body, so the more antioxidant protection we provide, the more stable it will be and the longer it will last. Doctors are utilizing this science by coating stents (mesh tubes that prop open arteries after surgery) with drugs that produce nitric oxide.

The side effect of poor blood flow is quite apparent to those over the age of 40. Older men tend to struggle with wound healing, hair loss, fatigue, certain types of memory loss and erectile dysfunction or ED.

During the course of my research, I discovered that beet roots contain a high concentration of dietary nitrates. Well you probably thought nitrites are bad for you. Nitrites are often used as an additive to hot dogs and meats and are known carcinogens when tested on lab rats. This form of nitrite is bad and should be avoided. Like cholesterol you have the good and the bad form in the body. The nitrates in beets are converted to a healthy form of nitrites in the body which can boost and stabilize nitric oxide in the blood.

Cardiovascular Benefits of Nitric Oxide
Maintain healthy blood pressure
Support normal triglyceride levels
Enhance healthy circulation
Promote artery health
Support cardiovascular and heart health
Improve exercise endurance and performance
Support sexual performance via improved circulations

Post Script:

In summary, the answer to the question, are you healthy enough for sex should to be addressed with patience and diligence by men. Use the information in this book to study and explore what works best for you. Keep in perspective that sex is our way of achieving immortality by leaving our DNA marker on this planet. Our very existence is the result of sex. The desire to live and survive is closely linked to our sex drive. Sex impacts many of the bodily systems such as the nervous system, circulatory, muscle, digestive function, and reproductive. Sex in general is best performed on an empty stomach or with at least a 2-4 hour window of digestion. Always avoid overeating. One would also be wise to skip the dessert or sweets several hours prior to sex to avoid insulin spikes. The saying goes when insulin goes up, testosterone comes down.

According to Chinese medicine, sugar in very yin and testosterone is very yang in function. Drinking too much alcohol can easily alter a man's yang nature into a more yin or weaken state. Both excess sugar and alcohol are not conducive for healthy vigorous sex. My best advice is to avoid drinking beer or any alcohol beverages prior to sex. The sugar content of beer or wine can also easily change a man's energy pattern to a yin state. Leave the sugar and alcohol alone when planning to have sex. Men should always try to pursue a healthy lifestyle. If you are a smoker then quit. Healthy sex is far more pleasurable than having a nicotine addiction.

According to the Chinese system of health, the element of water plays a crucial role. Water as an element relates directly to the kidney/bladder function. As you may recall, the kidneys are partially responsible for producing testosterone. Going to the gym, building muscles and playing sports targets the more external qualities of our health. The question is how healthy are your internal organs on the inside? What do you do for your sex organs? Just playing with it is not enough to maintain optimal functions and health.

Remember every individual situation is unique and requires solutions that are not always found within the confines of mainstream thought. Other topics on male sexuality will be presented and explored in my future books. I hope to make these upcoming books available to you soon.

References:

1. Shinde UA, Mehta AA, Goyal RK. Nitric Oxide: a molecule of the millennium. Indian J Exp Biol 2000 Mar:38(3): 201-10

2. Furchgott RF, Ignarro LJ, Murad F. Discover concerning nitric oxide as a signaling molecule in the cardiovascular system 1998. Nobel Prize in Medicine.

3. Guoyao W, Meininger CJ. Arginine Nutrition and Cardiovascular Function. J Nutr. 2000; 130: 2626-2629

4. Seidler M, Uckert S, Waldkirch E, Stief CG, Oelke M, Tsikas D, Sohn M, Jonas U. In vitro effects of a novel class of nitric oxide (NO) donating compounds on isolated human erectile tissue. Eur Urol. 2002 Nov;42(5):523-8

5. Taddei S, Virdis A, Ghiadoni L, Salvetti G, Bernini G, Magagna A, Salvetti A. Age-related reduction of NO availability and oxidative stress in humans,Hypertension(2001)Aug;38(2):274-9.

6. Guoyao WU, Morris SM. Arginine Metabolism: nitric oxide and beyond. Biochem J 1998; 336:1-17

7. Tomasian D, Keaney JF, Vita JA Antioxidants and the bioactivity of endothelium-derived nitric oxide. Cardiovasc Res. 2000 Aug 18;47(3):426-35.

8. Wollin SD, Jones PJ. Alpha-lipoic acid and cardiovascular disease. J Nutr. 2003 Nov;133(11):3327-30 Guoyao W, Meininger CJ. Arginine Nutrition Cardiovascular.   .

9. Elam RP, et al. Effects of Arginine and Ornithine on Strength, Lean Body Mass and Urinary Hydroxyproline in Adult Males. J Sports Med Phys Fitness. Mar1989;29 (1):52-56.

AFTER WORD

Am I healthy enough for sex is a question seldom asked by most men due to cultural expectation, male pride or self-denial? Most men naturally assume that the function and ability to have sex is their God given right and will happen without thought. In today's society such notions can no longer be considered the norm. This is largely due to our over exposure to synthetic estrogens, poor diet, obesity and limited arenas for expression of one's manhood.

What it means to be a man is constantly being defined and redefined. The new norms are ambiguous to many. The medical community keeps promising and selling us on a better sex life via Cialis and Viagra. The normal reference range for the average man's healthy testosterone level has declined significantly in the past 50 years. Our hormonal system has become more confused and unregulated by our body than ever in the history of man.

"Are You Healthy for Sex?" clearly highlights areas of concerns most men need to be aware of. Learn how you can offset hormonal decline and restore your body to optimal sexual health. Start making preparations now to revitalize your sex life with the knowledge presented in this book.

Dr. Angelo Isom ND, CHS, MQT

Visit my website for future updates, products and services. Phone/Skype consults are available by appointment. For detail information visit us at:

www.lifeishealing.com

www.harmonizingfist.com

Other books published by the author on sexual health and well being for men: "The Sexual Warrior Within" by Dr. Angelo Isom ND (Available at www.amazon.com)

Get my Free Report on

"8 Rare and Common Aphrodisiacs That Really Work"

Available on request at www.lifeishealing.com